Step Up

Your Present Situation Is Not Your Final Destination.

KEITH R. HARLEY, JR.

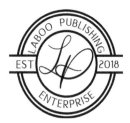

Table of Contents

Introduction

We often feel that where we come from, or our upbringing, has to dictate who we are! When we are children, we begin to form who we are as individuals at the age of three. We develop habits, we start to develop our personalities, we even form our sexuality. Our habits and behaviors are formed by our environment and our upbringing. Our beliefs are structured based on what we have been taught. Our level of confidence is determined by how we are treated and what we witness as children.

A simple hug, or a statement that says, "I love you," can give us a since of security, independence and confidence based on our surroundings and what they expose us to. These are the factors that will most profoundly determine our future unless we are courageous enough to conceptualize something different than our present situation.

Statistics say that your upbringing will determine your future. However, if you are exposed to different environments as you grow into adulthood, it will trigger curiosity to this other life that you have not been exposed to or experienced. Life has cycles, the beginning, the middle and the end.

In this book, *Step Up*, we will be talking about life experiences, and how these experiences affect your life and who you become. Do you like what you experienced in the beginning? Do you like what you're experiencing now, and what can you change so that at the end you will say to yourself, "Well done!"

This book will help you change your life based on experiences and not what you have been taught. It's time for you to Step Up, so that you can expose yourself beyond your present situation, find the potential, and be courageous enough to CHANGE, in all aspects of your life!

I am Keith Harley. I didn't like the beginning, where I came from. I am in the middle of my life, with the intent to be satisfied at the end. Let me tell you about my journey!

CHAPTER 1

I am Here
The Beginning of Life

I was born in Washington DC. My mother was Betty "Louise" Davis. She was a beautiful, brown-skinned woman with an amazing infectious smile. My dad was in the Navy, with striking features, an incredible smile and an amazing, friendly personality.

I don't remember much about my mom and dad's marriage because I was so young. However, I do remember the day that they made the decision to part ways. It was around the holidays. Even though I remember the sad feeling I had as a child when my dad decided to move on, I had no other choice but to understand—and I knew that I would see him again. When you have those experiences as a child, the pain you feel in the process, that is something you never forget.

What people don't realize is that those experiences as children go with us for the rest of our lives, whether they are pain, happiness or excitement. We never forget it, and as we become adults and go through life, there are certain experiences in our adulthood that will trigger those feelings we had as children. When we have those feelings, we can pretend like they don't exist or we can try to figure out why they are happening or why we are feeling this way. Nothing is more challenging than trying to figure out why we respond differently to different situations that have a negative impact on our feelings, moods and energy. Something can make us depressed, sad, unhappy and just downright sick, and we will never know why. Then as we get older, we start to watch other people's actions, and we begin to witness how others respond differently. We notice that the same thing will affect others in a way that is not the same when it comes to us.

I recall another unfortunate experience that I had as a child. I think I was about four or five. My mom took me to a babysitter. I remember this woman vaguely. She didn't live far from my mom's house. When my mom left me there, I remember the food she would serve me. Sometimes it was baloney sandwiches, or even Chef Boyardee. One day I remember watching TV. She grabbed me by the arm and took me to her bedroom. She laid me on the bed and blindfolded me. Now remember, I was about four or five years old. After she blindfolded me, I could feel her taking my clothes off. I could not really understand what was going on, however I knew something wasn't right. I laid there naked for some time, and then realized I was being touched—touched in a way that was unfamiliar to me. Touched in a way that I did not know how to respond. I didn't know whether to scream, yell or cry. I could see her out of the corner of the rag that she blindfolded me with. She was laying there naked, doing things to me that I felt were not right—or did I know it wasn't right? I was too young to understand. As far as I can remember, I didn't tell my mom or dad. I think that afterwards I just forgot about it. However, fast forward to today, and I remember all of it!

As I became older, my mom started dating a man who eventually became my stepfather. He was a good-looking man who took really good care of himself. He seemed to be really in love with my mom and treated her well. One day I will never forget, he brought over his dog to our small home in Maryland, not knowing that me and his dog would create a bond. Soon after, my mom and my stepdad decided to enjoy their lives together. My mom decided to start sending me to North Carolina to spend time with my grandmother.

Her name was Emma Belle Jamison. My grandmother was a sharp, spiritual, church-going woman who was a maid for some doctors in North Carolina.

I loved spending time with my grandmother, and I loved watching her prepare for church, as she wore these amazing hats and sang in the choir at a church called Hayes Memorial Baptist Church. The preacher's name was Bishop Fields. On Sunday mornings when my brother Anthony and myself would be with our grandmother, she would get up about 4:00am every morning and begin to cook our Sunday meal. She would always cook two meats, a rump roast and a chicken roast. She would also bake two cakes—one chocolate cake and one pound cake—from scratch. My grandmother could cook her butt off. Then, to add insult to injury, for breakfast she would fry chicken, and cook rice with gravy and homemade biscuits. I would wonder why she would get mad at me and my brother when we would go to church afterwards and fall asleep.

My experiences in Greensboro were sometimes amazing, and sometimes not. That's when I had my second experience that I did not understand and was not sure whether it was right. A family member began to touch me in ways that at that age I am sure were not right. I was again sexually abused over and over again for some years, and still did not understand whether it was right or wrong. It got to a point that it became regular for me and I thought it was something that I was supposed to do. I knew for some reason I could not tell my family members what was going on, or maybe I felt it was something you just didn't talk about, you just did it. You lay there and take it and you just don't talk about it. As I became older in my teens, this was still going on, not only from my family member, but also from a friend of the family! At this point, over the years I still had not told my mother. For some reason I had unspoken levels of fear. I didn't want to hurt my family and I sure did not want to hurt my mom, so I just took the pain of not understanding, I took the pain of thinking this was the right thing to do, and for years kept it to myself.

There were times that the family member and the friend of the family would say horrible, awful things to me before, during and after the sexual act. To this day I remember the names, the harsh tone in their voice and how hurt I felt afterwards. Even though I was young and was not understanding, I still had feelings. I guess this made these people feel in control. It made them feel bigger, it made them feel like they had control over me, which gave them power. But I still didn't understand. All I knew was that it was the right thing to do—or should I say I was thought and trained that it was what I was supposed to do.

Now, I did mention I have a brother. My mother did have a child before me. His name is Anthony Little. My brother and I never lived together. Anthony's father's mother adopted him when he was a baby and his grandmother cared for him as if he was her own. But Anthony and I would spend many summers together. It was so refreshing to have him around. You see, it would get lonely when it was just me and my mother! mother. My stepfather was around, however it was just so different when my brother was there. He protected me; when he was around, I didn't have those unwanted sexual advances from the family member or the friend of the family.

That is, until one hot summer night. I remember it was so hot in Greensboro, NC that we had box fans in the window. My uncle John and aunt Bee were in the house in the other room. They were asleep. Then it happened. It happened to me and my brother by these two family members. I was in shock; I was saddened and did not know how to talk to my brother about the incident. We just kept quiet. I could look in my brothers' eyes, he was so hurt. The family members that we looked up to did this to us, and he just could not understand. At this point he wanted to go home. He didn't want to be there any longer. Summers after that, he insisted on staying home and did not want to come and spend the summers with us. I could never understand, until now, when he was in his late 40s and I was in my early 40s, we discussed it, and then I finally understood why he was so distant.

Today, my brother and I are working on our relationship. He gets on me all the time about being closer, talking more, spending more time together, spending more time to get to know his family. You see, because of everything I went through as a child—the abuse, the hurt and the lack of attention—I did not know how to love, I didn't know how to cultivate lasting relationships.

After my mom and my stepdad divorced, it was just she and I. She had to work a lot to keep a roof over our head. She didn't let her circumstances hold her back from getting out there and making things happen, she did what she had to do to make ends meet. So the lack of attention as a child and a teenager did not allow me to develop those relationship skills. I thought relationship skills were being abused and hurt, so I just didn't understand. As you get older and you begin to watch others and their families, you begin to ask yourself, "Why didn't I have those experiences?" You ask yourself, "What is wrong with me?" So as you're watching, you're noticing people are happier. They do things for themselves that make them happy. They are respected. They have tough skin and they relate to other people differently. You notice they are not people pleasers. You see, when you're abused, especially at a young age, you think the best way to get people to love you is to please them in any way you can. You're always thinking, "Does this person like me, do they want to talk to me, do they want to be my friend," and so on. Then when you realize they could care less, your heart is broken. When you're older and you can't please the people that are around you, you feel the same pain you felt when you were abused. This is not easy to change. You first have to understand it before you can change it! It's hard work, but once you understand it, your energy begins to shift. You become more confident, you have thicker skin and you don't settle for things that are not of you. You begin to get your POWER. It's a feeling that I can't explain, but it's WONDERFUL.

Remember, it's a process and it takes time. You even at times need professional help, but trust me, when you get it, you become FREE!

CHAPTER 2

I Knew it was Wrong, but Did I Have a Choice?

Once I decided that I wanted to understand why I was the way I was, I knew I needed to find out how and what I could do about it. One day I was with a client and she told me she was seeing a psychiatrist, and that her life had changed since she had been seeing this woman. I thought to myself, I want to go. I want to learn about me and who I am and why. So I made an appointment, I showed up, and walked into her beautiful home. She was exquisite, she was classy, she spoke with such authority and grace. Let's just call her Dr. W.

Dr. W asked me several questions to get to know me. She made me feel right at home and was an amazing listener! I felt, for the first time ever, that I was free and able to speak the truth without being judged. It was almost like she could relate and she was truly interested in what I had to say. She was not shocked about my life, and at the end she told me I was the way I was not because I wanted to be, but because it was what I had been taught. She also told me I had to forgive the others, forgive myself and rebirth myself so that I could live the life I deserved and desired. She told me I was not a mistake, but I was a blessing, and that what I had been through I had to accept. It was time to rebirth myself. It was time that I confronted my fears head on and moved beyond where I had been stuck in my life. She made me realize it was not a choice what happened to me. I was a child, I didn't understand, and those things that happened to me were not my choice, they were someone's else's. I was just the victim. At this point in my life, I could no longer be the victim, I had to become the victor. I had to become the man I was supposed to be and I had to make a change. This was a long process and not an easy one, but I did it!

When you center yourself around people that inspire you to do better, inspire you to be better and inspire you to level up, you have no other choice but to address your fears, confront your past and work on becoming a better you! If you don't address the issues that are holding you back, you will never have the opportunity to grow yourself, and at the end, you will never sing your song because it will be too late! I know it's easier to say it than to do it. However, if you push through the pain and fear, you will be happy about the results, and the ton of bricks that you have been carrying will be knocked off. As time went on, I continued my therapy. I began to realize that the way I was living my life was a reflection of my past. I realized that the only way that I would change my life or even know that there was a possibility was exposure to something different. Something different than I had ever seen. So moving forward, I started hanging in a friend's salon. I observed and watched, and then, as time went on, I started working in a salon as a cleaning person. That didn't last long. One night, I was cleaning and I left some towels in the utility sink. When we turned on the washing machine and the water began to drain, the towels clogged the sink. Then the water came out of the sink and began to flood the whole salon. To add insult to injury, one of the stylists came into work, didn't see the water, slipped and sprained her ankle! Needless to say I was fired that day. As time went on, I didn't give up. I knew the beauty industry was for me. I just didn't know what my calling and my gift was— but it sure wasn't cleaning the salon.

One day I went to get my hair done. I would go to the salon and get a perm, you probably know it as a Jerri curl, the proper term is perm. As I was watching my stylist Sheila do my curl, I realized I could learn to do this myself. This is what she would do: straighten, curl and neutralize. I would watch her do this every time I would get my hair done. I said, "I can do this," so I went to the store with $2.50 and I bought myself a *RightOn Magazine*. I cut out some pictures, glued them to a clean white piece of paper, and I wrote on the paper, "Curls for $35."

Moving forward that was my daily job, while my mom was at work. Between the hours of 3:00pm and 6:00pm I would do curls in the basement of my mom's home. She didn't know it. By the time she would get home, I would have all of the clients done and out of the house and the house was clean smelling like Pine-sol. One day, I was in the basement working hard: curls flowing, dryers moaning and the TV was on, and the clients were watching Ms. Chancellor on *The Young and the Restless*. I was rolling a curl and I thought I heard the door charm ring, which means someone walked in the front door. Now one thing I knew for sure is that no one walked in the door without knocking, and the only one that had the privilege was my mom, and that was because she owned the place.

The next thing I heard was a loud screeching voice yelling, "CORKEYYYY!" Corkey was my mom's nickname for me. I ran upstairs. She was standing at the top of the steps, and she said, "Whose cars are in the driveway and why can't I get in my garage?" I froze and was speechless, I didn't know what to say. Mom pushed me out of the way, walked down the steps and saw eight women sitting in the basement—which smelled like rotten eggs, by the way, because anyone that has ever had a perm done knows that's the worst smell in the world. My mom looked at the basement, then looked at me, and said, "What in the world is going on and who are these women in my house? Get them out right now!"

I said, "But Mom..."

She said, "Now!"

I said, "You don't understand," as I was following her up the steps. Once we arrived up the stairs and I followed her in the kitchen, I said, "Mom, please."

She said, "Corkey, I have told you, no company in the house when I am not home without my permission. You know I work hard every day to keep a roof over our head, and all I ask of you is to do your homework, keep the house clean and have no company when I am not in the house."

I put my head down, with this sad face, and began to think about crying, because the last thing I wanted to do was disappoint my mother. That's how I was then and that is how I am now. I never want to disappoint anyone. I wanted you to love me, be my friend and like me, that was because I was a pleaser, which stemmed from my abuse as a child. So I looked at my pockets, and I noticed they were full. I reached in and pulled a wad of money out of my pocket that I made that week. I raised my hand and showed it to my mom, and said to her, "What do I do with this?"

She looked at my hand, looked at me, then looked at my hand with the money, then looked at me again and said, "I will be right back." The next thing you know, my mom came in the kitchen with an apron on. She said, "Do they want some Mac and cheese, greens, corn bread, homemade biscuits and some fried chicken?" My mom saw that money and it was on.

I did not know at that moment I was becoming an entrepreneur! It seemed to come so naturally, but then I realized later in life that my mom always had the entrepreneurial spirit. She owned stores, businesses and much more. I guess watching her gave me some insight on who I wanted to be in the future. Later I started incorporating other services for my customers into my business. I started an image consulting business at the age of 17. I always had an eye for fashion and loved clothes. I loved watching my grandmother getting dressed, especially when she was going to church, the way she wore her hat, her shoes and her dresses. My grandmother always took pride in how she carried herself. In those days, our grandparents understood the importance of dressing well, showing others that when you take pride in the way you look, it increases your self-esteem, confidence and image. It makes me wonder whether my love for the beauty industry comes from watching my mother and grandmother so often.

I even considered going to Barbizon Modeling School. That was interesting. When I met with the representative at the school, I didn't realize she would tell me everything that was wrong with me in order for me to go to the school. She even made me stand against the wall. She said that if there was a gap between my back and the wall, that meant that I had bad posture. Can you imagine what that did to my self-esteem as a teenager? So needless to say, I didn't attend that school. I later attended a modeling school that was much more affordable. The owner of the school was absolutely amazing. Her name was Misty. She instilled so much in me, confidence, love and attention. My instructor's name at the school was Terri Washington. He modeled for Fashion Fair and other major modeling companies, not to mention a lot of magazines and ads. Terri showed me how to walk, talk, and dress. He became like a mentor and a big brother to me. When Terri walked in, he would command a room with his confidence and swagger. I knew I wanted to be just like him.

Fast forward, I was still trying to find myself. I was trying to figure out who I wanted to be and what I wanted to do. It was a bit difficult to figure out what was the wrong way or the right way. My mother was constantly working, making sure we had a roof over our head. I didn't get a chance to see my dad much, so I was often alone. My mother tried so hard to make us have a normal home. At times it was difficult and a strain on her, but she always seemed to make a way. She had a strong constitution and she didn't take any mess! I didn't know much about my mom's upbringing; she really didn't talk much about it. I never met my grandfather on my mom's side but I did have the pleasure of meeting my dad's father, William Harley. He was a quiet storm. The only time I would see him is when I went to my father's family house. My grandad was always upstairs in his bedroom in the bed with fresh clean pajamas. It seems like he never came out of that room. I remember his pure white hair and his white beard. Later on my dad told me that my grandfather worked for the government and that he worked for years without taking a sick day or time off. His work ethic was incredible.

As a child, I witnessed so much, not realizing how all of these experiences would affect me as an adult. My mom was an entrepreneur, my dad served in the Navy and worked extremely hard and was so nice. I really think I got my personality from my dad. He loved people, he loved to help people, and he would give you the shirt off his back. Later in life he married my stepmom. She was a bit younger than him and had an amazing head on her shoulders. We bonded from day one. I will never forget the day I met her. She looked at me, I looked at her and could not help but notice how incredibly nice she was. To this day she calls me son. When I hear her and my dad say son, my heart just melts. I am getting a little teary-eyed writing this. One thing a child at any age yearns for is love and attention, they want to feel like they belong. I think as a child I was alone so much, and suffering from sexual abuse, so I just wanted some type of connection with my parents. I would see other children with their parents and the relationships they had as a family. I wanted that so much, but I understood why I couldn't.

My mom did remarry and I had a stepdad. He was a good guy. I truly cared for him. However, as time went on, my mom and stepdad had some issues and things just didn't work out. Sometimes in the home was very uncomfortable, the arguing, fussing and fighting and not to mention the sexual abuse that was happening right under their noses. Those years were tough, and at times took a toll on my mom, to the point that being in the house was difficult. One night I couldn't take it anymore so I ran away from home. I had a grown-up friend pick me up down the street from my mom's house. I went to his house and called my dad. Lord, what did I do that for? My dad did not play. He came right away and I was scared for me and my friend who picked me up, because my dad did not know what was going on. Once my dad picked me up, the following day we had a conversation about me going to military school. At the time I thought it was a good idea, because I just wanted to get away from home into a different environment. A couple of days later my dad took me home. It was a bit uncomfortable, because my mom was disappointed in me and my dad had to go. My dad never yelled at me, he never stayed upset with me and even when he knew I was wrong, he never made me feel that he would not forgive me. See even though me and my dad never lived together, and I knew that he had gone on with his life, I always had this deep love for him. He was my dad and I knew he could only do what he knew how and what he was capable of doing. I didn't understand then, but I understand now. Today I am doing everything in my power to call him more and spend more time with him. I try to let him know that I love him dearly, and despite the lost time, the distance and the lack of communication, I know it was not all his fault. I know he could do only what he was allowed, and I am forever grateful that he is my dad. DADDY, I LOVE YOU! Always know I truly believe that you are an incredible, strong man and you inspire me to be happy, live an amazing life and treat others with kindness.

The sexual abuse I experienced during my childhood conditioned my mind as an adult to be a people pleaser. I had low self-esteem and no self-worth. I constantly wore my heart on my sleeve. I took everything to heart, as if everyone was out to hurt me. All I wanted was to be loved. As I became older, mentally I was still a little boy. I could act like an adult in some cases, but really in my head I was a little boy that wanted to be loved. Interestingly enough, I thought this was normal, because I was not exposed to anything different. I didn't know right from wrong, I just lived based on what I experienced as a child.

The side effects I had as an adult from my childhood were that I was nervous all the time and scared. I was always rushing, even when I went to the bathroom—I even thought doing that was shameful. I was always breaking stuff, hurting myself, being clumsy, having accidents, dropping things, shaking, wetting the bed, not remembering things, having a hard time in school. It was difficult to develop relationships and friendships—and the list goes on. Then I realized I had to address these issues and fix them, because as I began to expose myself to other environments, I knew there was a better way of living, so I changed my circle of influence. I started hanging around those that I wanted to be like, to the point I lied about my age so that I could work, hang around older people and learn all over again. One of the things that I have learned is that my past does not equal my future. Someone once said, "You will never change what you're not willing to acknowledge." When you acknowledge your past and you realize that you want to change, you begin to seek out what you may think is better for you. In the quest of trying to figure out what is best for you, you never know the difference between right and wrong.

People will take advantage of you when they know you are seeking help to change your life. When you have a past like mine, all you want to do is please everybody, not realizing that some people are just not good for you. Between the ages of 20 and 40, I had to learn the hard way, I wanted everyone to be my friend, I wanted to be liked, loved, and accepted. This type of behavior was not good for a young man who wanted to be successful in the business world. I learned later that was a form of weakness and people in the business world would eat me for lunch.

As I took on many jobs, it was difficult to keep them, because my low self-esteem would get the best of me. I remember one job in particular. I worked for a temp agency called Kelly Temps and they sent me to IBM in Bethesda, Maryland to be a receptionist. When I showed up for work that morning at 7:45am, 15 minutes early, I remember checking in at the desk and the young lady going to get the human resources manager to come and get me to show me around. The women came out, looked at me and said hello. Then she told me she would be back to get me. Four hours passed; she never came back. I finally called my temp manager at Kelly's Temps and told her I had been sitting there for four hours and she replied, "What? I'll call you right back." An hour later, after sitting in the waiting room for 5 hours, she called me back and said, "They will not be needing your services today." I knew the moment I saw that women she didn't like me just based on the way I looked. I guess I didn't fit the image that IBM was looking for at that time. You can imagine how I felt walking out of that building and going home. I felt rejected, hurt and judged. Let's be clear: if my self-esteem was at a higher level, none of that would have bothered me, BUT I was already broken and I didn't know how to practice emotional management. I didn't even know how to process different thinking, and especially thinking about myself.

In my 30s and 40s I realized that things like this affected me as an adult. When people would treat me a certain way or say certain things to me that felt hurtful and uncomfortable, it would remind me of who I used to be as a child. Oftentimes if you don't confront those issues as a child, they will stay with you until you become an adult, which would make you very sensitive, and give you low confidence and low self-esteem.

How many of you ever wonder why you are so different from everybody else, why you are so sensitive, why you are so receptive to having your feelings hurt, and having them smoothed over again so easily? That is because how we are brought up, or the experiences we've had as children, stick with us throughout our adulthood. But as I stated on the cover of this book, *your present situation is not your final destination*.

If you want to fix who you are today, take the Band-Aid off and heal the wounds of your past. When you start to do that, you will look at some of the things that happened to you as a child and then you will think to yourself, Oh my God, is that where that is from? Once you do that, I want you to remember to look back and go back to who you used to be to remind yourself how far you've come. But you have to remember not to stay there. People will have a tendency to stay there because that's what's comfortable for them.

The hard work is moving forward, and you have to be able to work on yourself every day to take yourself out of your past. Let me be clear: when you begin to change yourself, people remind you of who you used to be, because that is what's comfortable for them. But you have to be courageous enough to keep moving forward. It's going to seem lonely in the process, but that is just God clearing your path to receive your blessing that is deserved to you. So my question for you is: are you ready for the process of change? Are you willing to do the work? Understand that it's not going to happen overnight. But if you work hard every day, I promise you, you will be excited about the results. You will be able to wake up every morning with a smile, energy, and ready to tackle the world with confidence, high self-esteem and an ability to interact with all types of people that come your way. We often complain about the results we didn't get because of the work we didn't do, so do the work and be unapologetic, intentional and focused.

Let me give you a few examples of the steps that you take to create change in your life:

- Acknowledge the pain
- Get professional help
- Do the work
- Don't give up on yourself
- Don't stop until the work is done
- Stay away from the naysayers in the process of change
- Be OK with leaving people behind

I promise you, once you began to do the work on yourself things will began to change in your life.

CHAPTER 3

The Habits Begin to Form

As I stated before, in the beginning of this book, between the ages of three and 16 is when your life begins to form. Your life is developed based on how you were treated as a child. But most importantly, you have to make a decision that your past does not equal your future and, again, that your present situation is not your final destination. Some people don't understand that as you get older you have to decide what is right and what is wrong. How you do that is to expose yourself to a different environment. You have to want something more for yourself. However, doing that means you have to confront some issues and understand that if you want a different life you have to have exposure, because sometimes, we don't know that a different life is available to us. We always make the excuse that where we are from or how we are brought up determines how we have to be, and that is not true at all. One thing I remember from when I was a little boy was my mother taking me to the babysitter. When my mother would go off to work, I remember that this particular babysitter would sit me down with the rest of the kids at the kitchen table. One thing that I remember is hearing the sound of *The Young and the Restless* or *One Life to Live*, shows that were on TV at the time. Then the babysitter would grab my hand and walk me to her bedroom. Once I got to her bedroom, she would blindfold me. Once she would blindfold me, she would lay me on her bed and I couldn't see anything but pitch-black darkness. However, I still remember listening to the sounds of the TV shows that were on the TV. I would be laying on the bed and then I would realize nothing was going on for about the first 5 to 10 minutes. Then I remember this large body hovering over me, touching me inappropriately, and at the time I didn't know what it was. I didn't know who it was, but I later realized that it was my babysitter, and she was molesting me. I remember being about three years old or maybe four years old, and certain details of this awful experience remain vivid. This is one of the examples of how events that happen to you as a child can impact your life. As I'm sitting here writing this, I am realizing that it happened on more than one occasion with more than one person. It happened with another babysitter and it also happened with a family member.

As I reflect on these unfortunate circumstances in my past as a child, today I realize how my past had a true effect on me and my self-esteem and my lack of confidence. I grew up wanting to be loved, wanting to have friends and feeling like I needed someone in my life to make my life complete. When you're a child you don't realize that this is not normal. It becomes your normal, and your mind has been conditioned to think this is OK, that this is the way people show love. And all of this time my mother and my dad never knew. I suppressed it, and as I grew older, I didn't have the heart to have a discussion with them when I became a teenager. As I said, I didn't know what was right from wrong, I didn't know if this was the wrong thing to do or if it was the right thing to do, and whether it was acceptable. All I knew was that it happened to me many times and I could never understand why. Why was I the chosen one to experience all of this, why was I the one to be molested over and over again from a young baby boy? To this day I still don't understand it, but I'm grateful that I received the help that I needed to become the man that I am today.

You have to allow yourself the opportunity to understand what is right and what is wrong. You first have to realize that you cannot blame yourself, and then you have to forgive, so that you won't have hate in your heart for the rest of your life. Because if you don't get help, it's a possibility that hate is what you're going to feel.

Once you determine what is right or wrong and you get some help, you have to start taking care of yourself and realizing that you are either a boy or girl interrupted. What I mean by that is, as children our lives were interrupted by these unfortunate circumstances. Now some of us still may have the mindset of a little boy or a little girl, but at some point, we have to grow up and we have to say to ourselves, "I'm an adult now, and what has happened in my past is no longer a part of me," and each and every day you have to work hard at it.

If you were abused, or mentally scarred for any given reason, you have the opportunity to fix it. You need to take your Band-Aid off your wound, let it heal, and sometimes you need a little bit of medicine, to get some help, but that's okay. You should not have to suffer any longer for what you went through in your past as a child.

I have so many stories that I could share with you from when I was a child. Statistics would tell you, based on what I've been through, I should be an emotional wreck, but I can tell you I'm good, because I did the work. There were many times in my life that I would rush through doing things, and never have the full experience, because I would think it would either be embarrassing, I wasn't doing it right, or someone would criticize me. I would find myself shaking doing the most insignificant things or being nervous. Even going to the restroom, I used to rush just to go pee because I didn't want people to even hear me or know what I was doing. Let's not forget that, as a child in my teenage years, my nerves were so bad based on what I was experiencing, I used to pee in the bed. Do you know how embarrassing that was? My mother would get so upset with me and I would try to hide it, but at certain points I couldn't even hide it anymore. She would eventually find out.

I remember when my mom and my stepfather used to go out in the evenings and my stepfather insisted that it was time for me to learn how to stay home alone. I must've been 10 or 11, I can't remember, but when they would go out, I literally would lock myself in the bedroom and hide under the bed until my mom and stepdad came home. Sometimes I would fall asleep, and my mom and dad would get upset because they couldn't get into the room, because I had barricaded the door hoping and praying that no one would come in while they were gone.

One night in particular I was home in my bedroom reading on the floor. My mom and stepdad were in the next room and then, all of a sudden, I heard this big boom and it literally came through my bedroom window. Someone had thrown a brick through my bedroom window. That was the kind of bullying I experienced when I was in elementary school. It was pure torture, and I couldn't understand why people would want to do that to me. I would always ask, why me?

My mom was always the aggressive one in the relationship between my stepdad and her, so of course when the brick came through the window she was pissed off, and she ran outside to find out who did it. My stepdad stayed inside looking out of the window, and I looked up at him wondering, "What are you going to do to protect me?" Many times my mother had to come out of the house and protect me from the neighborhood bullies. My mom played the role of my mother and my father at times. She was not afraid of anything, but interestingly enough, I was afraid of everything. I think at some point she was trying to figure out why I was always so afraid of people, and why I was always walking around afraid. It made her very upset because she didn't understand. However, when you are a child and all these things have happened to you, it's difficult to express yourself or tell your mom or dad what is going on with you.

In the culture that I was from, we would never discuss the things that happened to me, that was just the way it was. I'm sure some of you can relate. In our culture all we would do was just suffer through the consequences and hope that we would turn out okay. My mom always used to tell me, "What goes on in our house stays in our house." We would never discuss our business outside of the house, and we were never to embarrass our family. This was the rule, and if you broke the rule you would get in major trouble. It wasn't about what happened to you, it was about what was shared outside of the household. It was almost like you were trapped, whatever you did. If you tried to express yourself you would get in trouble; and if you kept your mouth shut you would get in trouble, because you would act out in other ways due to the reflection of what you had been through.

If you're a parent and you're reading this, pay attention to the actions of your children. They may be trying to tell you something and not know how to verbalize it.

I can give you a prime example. When my mother thought that there was something wrong with me mentally or there was something wrong with me sexually, she took me to her doctor and she said, "There's something wrong with my son and I need you to fix him." At that very moment I was confused, embarrassed and trying to understand why my mother did that, not realizing that she had her own issues that she was dealing with and it was very hard for her to accept what was going on with me at the time. She didn't know who to turn to, she didn't know who to talk to, she just wanted to get it right, without really understanding the full details. And she could not understand the full details because I could not express to her what I had been through over the years, so our relationship in the beginning was extremely difficult.

Finally, when I went to high school, I couldn't even relate to my classmates because mentally I was already beyond what a teenager or a child should be like, because I already had experienced adult activities. To make a long story short, my childhood was interrupted. I never had the opportunity to live as a kid the way that a normal child should. I had adult activities from the age of three on up, so I was always living in fear, trying to please people, and worried about whether people liked me or not.

Why did I worry about whether people liked me or not? Because when you have those experiences of molestation as a child, people do what they want to you, treat you bad, and then get up and leave you. I remember a couple of incidents that I can relate to why I was always afraid of abandonment. After one session of me being molested, when this person finished their sexual act with me, they looked at me and said, "Look at you. You're just a little faggot and that's what you will always be." Another time when a person molested me, when they finished their sexual act, they had soiled their clothes, so they turned around and punched me in my chest so hard I lost consciousness and couldn't breathe. When I woke up, they asked me, "Why did you let this get on my pants?" Then I was told to get out of there and get away from them, and I was called some names. I can't remember in particular what names but I knew they were awful.

At the time this was going on my mother was literally downstairs with some friends. Again, like I told you, I was afraid to tell her what was going on, and I didn't think she would believe me. I was afraid to hurt my mom and I was afraid to tell on him, the person that was doing it, because I thought they would do something to hurt me. That's where the confusion came. I didn't know the difference between right and wrong.

After that moment in time my mom and my stepfather decided to divorce. They were not getting along and my stepfather decided to move on with his life. That was extremely difficult for me, because my real father left when I was three years old on Christmas Day. So at some point I thought that my stepfather, who my mother met when I was five, was going to step in and be that father figure to me. But it didn't work out that way, so again me and my mom were left alone.

It was extremely difficult when my stepdad left. It was financially difficult and emotionally difficult. I think my mom was mentally drained. I was told as a young child that my mother suffered a nervous breakdown. I was sent to Greensboro, North Carolina to spend months with my grandmother and my aunt Bea, not knowing that my mother was going through so much while I was home in the country. We had lost our home and had foreclosed, and she had lost her business. As a matter fact, she had two businesses. One was a bookkeeping service called Davis and Davis and Associates, and she had two convenience stores. My mom was a true entrepreneur and I truly believe that's where I got my entrepreneurial spirit from.

One day I was at school and I fell down and I fractured my arm. The school called my mom and told her I had hurt myself and my arm was swollen. My aunt Pam came to school to pick me up because my mother was still at work. I always loved when my mom or my aunt came to the school, because at that time, we had this beautiful Pontiac Firebird that was sky blue. When people would see that beautiful sky bird come around the corner, they would go absolutely crazy and it just did something to me to see my mom come to my school when she could. It wasn't often because she was a hard worker so she didn't have that opportunity. But one thing I must say, when my mom couldn't show up, my aunt Pam did! One thing about my aunt Pam was she always knew how to make me feel good when my mother or my stepdad were not available or they were out working. My favorite meal that she would fix would be white sticky rice with corn. I don't know what it was about the rice and corn mixed together. I guess it was the love that she would put in it.

Now interestingly enough my aunt Pam was not really my aunt, she was my stepdad's niece, and she came into my family by marriage, so I'm assuming she was my cousin in law. But from the first day that she came into my life she was always that solid person that didn't do anything to hurt me. She always showed me love and always supported me in anything that I did. Pam is everything to me, and the more successful

I become, I will always make sure she has the life that she has always wanted. It has always been my goal and always will be! I can't wait for the opportunity to take her on a vacation or put her in an incredible home that she can call her own. I owe that to her. During times when my mom and my stepdad were working really hard and they weren't home, and some other things that were going on that I wasn't aware of that I would later find out, or when they weren't getting along, my aunt Pam would always show me the love that I needed and I am forever grateful to her for that.

So back to the story. She picked me up from school. My arm was swollen and my mother had to finish a project before she took me to the hospital. When she took me to the hospital, they told me I had fractured my arm and I needed a cast, but unfortunately, I could not get a hard cast. They had to give me a soft cast, because we did not have the proper insurance to get the hard cast. They gave me a soft wrap around my arm and we had to pray that my arm was going to heal correctly, and I thank God that my arm did heal correctly. To this day, they said that was a miracle. I couldn't explain to you why that happened, but after that I never had any issues with my arm again.

The lesson behind this experience was that I had to deal with the fact that I couldn't get the proper care, because we were in a bad situation and there was nothing we could do about it. At that point I felt like it was my fault, and I didn't want to add any more problems to my mother's plate than she already had. I could see the frustration on her face and my heart hurt so bad to see my mother upset, but we got past that moment and we moved on. There were many instances like that. Those are just a few that I can remember. I was having these major experiences as a child in adult situations. I had to be emotionally stern so that I could support my mom through that situation

As you're reading this, you're probably saying, "Wow, that was a lot!" I will tell you it was. I was a child that had to be an adult and I had to emotionally support my mother through her trials and tribulations. I had to deal with molestation, abuse, being bullied and the emotional stress of supporting my mother through her setbacks. I also had to be the person that had to take the effects of bad situations adults had to go through, and I had to suffer the consequences for things that I had nothing to do with.

If you suffered any situations of this kind as a child, this may be the reason why as an adult you suffer from low self-esteem, lack of confidence and always feeling nervous. And you're trying to figure out what is the difference between right and wrong in the actions of others and how they benefit you or how they take you down. It's almost like you have to rebirth yourself and learn all over again: learn how to be a child, learn how to enjoy life, learn how to take your time, learn how to enjoy every moment and not be nervous. Often, when you're in the midst of living your life and being happy, you become uncomfortable, because happiness is not familiar to you so you look for something to always be wrong. You need to realize that when there's nothing wrong, it's okay,

You have to give yourself permission to get to a clear understanding of what the difference is between right and wrong, and it's okay. Be patient with yourself, tell yourself it's going to be okay, and take one day at a time. When you do it this way, I guarantee you will be okay.

CHAPTER 4

Who Do You Go to for Help?

Who do you go to for help? That's a good question. As a child, I had no idea that help even existed.

The definition of help: 1. Verb: make it easier for (someone) to do something by offering one's services or resources 2. Noun: the action of helping someone to do something; assistance.

So often you think to yourself, I need help, what do I do? But then I realized, I didn't even know how help existed. I started watching other people, looking at how they lived their lives, and I started to vicariously live through them. But most importantly, at some point, I had to realize that that was not going to work for the rest of my life. I had to make my dreams my reality, and the first step was to help myself and change who I was based on what I experienced in the past. That was a very hard thing to do, to go back and relive my past. You have to leave some of the things behind but some of the things you can take with you.

As I'm writing this book I keep starting and stopping, starting and stopping, and the reason for that is, as I began to relive my past, it was very difficult to complete this project. Dealing with emotions, disappointments, the loss of my mother, re-developing a relationship with my family, and the list goes on and on. I was not making any excuses, I was just truly overwhelmed with emotion during this process, but I'm grateful that I was able to go back and gain some understanding.

It is vitally important to realize that you need help. The second thing is you have to identify the problems that you need help with. Then, as you begin to reach out to people you trust, you need to let them know that you have a goal for change, and that you want them to be a part of the change, to support you.

For me the process of getting to know people and to trust them is, they have to prove themselves. You cannot always accept people into your life immediately. I always tell people: You have to put yourself back in the glass case and take yourself off the sale rack. What I mean by that is, you need to teach people how to treat you. That process allows you to get to know people. Don't always be so gullible as to let people in. You never know if there's a hidden motive, if they're genuine or if they're trustworthy.

When you begin to teach people how to treat you, it frees you up from being disappointed, or diminishing the value of who you are in your existence. A lot of people don't understand that. We do it backwards. We become people pleasers. We think that's the first step of establishing our relationship, friendship, or whatever. That is not how it goes. Based on my past and being affected by sexual abuse, that is what made me very passive, afraid, and always looking for validation. When you are a victim of sexual abuse, there's certain traits you take with you as a child to an adult. You think it is your job to please others and to accept anybody in your life to fill a void, because that's what you've been accustomed to: someone coming and taking advantage of you; and after they do what they came to do, they get up and leave you and treat you like you're an option.

Can you imagine being a child going through these unfortunate circumstances and you have no choice because you're a child? Then you grow up, and you have to deal with all of those things that you experienced as an adult. And that's how you continue to live your life until you realize what the problems are and you begin to work to fix them.

I'm here to tell you, yes, these things can be fixed, and yes, you can change your life. But it takes work and it takes getting around people who understand you, who understand your past and are non-judgmental. Once you find these people, that's when the work begins, because these are people that are not going to allow you to fail. These are the people that are going to hold you accountable, they are not going to let you stop. They're going to hold you up when you fail or fall. Those are the people that you want in your inner circle, who are going to support you through this process of change during the healing from your past.

Now let's talk about being judgmental. Some people are going to hear your story and they're going to be extremely judgmental, and usually the people who are judgmental are the ones who have not had these types of experiences. But because of who you are, you initially will feel like someone has dismissed you or they don't value your relationship or your friendship. But you need to understand people cannot talk about nor do anything about something that they have not experienced or been taught, and with that being said, you can't take anything personal. You can't be upset or disappointed, just focus on the healing and the work that comes with it.

There is one very important thing that you need to understand. There's an old saying my mother used to say to me all the time: What goes on in this house stays in this house. Now that's to an extent, let's be clear. Most importantly, you have to understand you have to choose the right people to open up to about your past and the situations that you are dealing with. Not everybody has that privilege, and that is the first thing you need to understand in this process. Not everyone has the privilege to be in your personal space, because when you expose your past, your situations and your issues that you're dealing with, that makes you vulnerable and people will take advantage of that. So be very careful who you expose your past to, and the things that you're working on. As my good friend Gloria Mayfield-Banks always says, guard your circle of influence, it is imperative.

There was a time that I would tell people about my past and certain things that I'd been through, and some of those people disappointed me, because they took my information and they used it to talk about me or to devalue my existence. So when I would find out that they were either gossiping or spreading my personal business, it was hurtful, and that's when I had to realize that hurt people hurt people. With that being said, I realized that I could not expose myself to just any and everybody, and you have to do the same thing.

Do you know our heritage, and how prideful our generations were about personal business? You did not want to embarrass your family or disappoint your parents, so generationally, that was something that was at the top of the list. You did not break the family code, and if you did, you would suffer for it, because your aunties, your uncles, and your cousins would let you know that you were at fault for exposing your personal information or the family's personal information, which would be embarrassing the family. Generationally, that was the rule.

However, now that we're in a different time in the world, oftentimes when you expose certain things, that's when change begins to happen. So don't ever allow people, family members, or friends to criticize you for being open about your problems and your situation. Yet, at the same time, be mindful with who you tell and who you give that privilege to.

Let me tell you, as I have spoken about this earlier in this book, it is okay to seek professional help. Again, generationally, that was not what we did from my culture, but the way things are done now, it's acceptable to get professional help. There are some people more equipped than you that can help you with the mental stuff that you're dealing with. It's okay to go to someone for understanding, a plan, and to do the work and assist you with it. Don't let the generational actions make you feel guilty for the actions that you're about to take for change.

Honestly, this was one of the reasons why I was reluctant about writing this book, because I was afraid of the people who abused me mentally and physically. To this day, at the age of 54, I still walk around with fear of these people and what they would do to me if I exposed what I experienced as a child. But I would be doing myself and other people a disservice. There are other people that are suffering from what I've suffered, and I want them to know that they can be free from it and they can begin the work and not walk in fear.

The definition of fear to me is *False Evidence Appearing Real*. We always make our decisions based on the fear that we've had and the conversations that we have in our head. No longer will you or I walk in fear, no longer will we allow our past to keep us quiet. It is time to stand up, get the help that you need, change your life and move forward. One most important thing I want you to always understand is, do not go to your grave in regret. Grab life by the balls, fix your stuff and begin to live right now.

CHAPTER 5
Understanding the Habits

hab·it /ˈhabət/ noun 1. 1. a settled or regular tendency or practice, especially one that is hard to give up. "we stayed together out of habit."

The word habit most often refers to a usual way of behaving or a tendency that someone has settled into, as in "good eating habits." In its oldest sense, however, habit meant "clothing" and had nothing to do with the things a person does in a regular and repeated way.

So we now understand the word habit, and over time I had to realize what a habit was. I had always been told that the definition of a habit is something that we do for 21 days over time, and it becomes something regular in our lives. One of the things that I've learned over time is there's a difference between a habit and a lifestyle. In my speaking and teachings, I always say you don't want to create a habit; you want to create a lifestyle. 21 days is not long enough, so I tell people to take 90 days to create a lifestyle, because 21 days is short term. Anything that you want to change in your life, give yourself 90 days to do it consistently on a daily basis, and then it will become a lifestyle.

A lot of the habits that I have today are a reflection of what I've been through as a child and a young adult. Some of the habits are good and some of the habits are bad, but with work the bad habits can be changed, and with that change I can incorporate new and good habits so that I can sustain an amazing, happy life, and I won't go back to who I used to be.

People often do not realize what the habit is, because they think that is their way of living and it's okay. A lot of people always make the excuse, "This is the way I was brought up," "That is where I'm from," or, "This is just the way that I am." Some people don't identify or know if their habit is even wrong, just because of the way that they were brought up, with the way that they were treated by their parents or family members or outside friends. So it's important that we identify what the habits are and understand if the habits are good. Once we establish that, we have to make an effort to understand the habits and begin to change some of those habits that are not good. No more making excuses. Listen to what people tell you, what they experience with you. That is usually an indication that there is a change that needs to be made. In that process your habits will become a lifestyle and you will incorporate that into your success of happiness and understanding.

There's not a lot to talk about in this chapter about habits because it's simple and it's straight to the point. You just have to understand what those habits are.

How do you change habits? Follow the steps below:

1: Identify your habits: Do a self-inventory of who you are, how you do things, how your relationships are, and friendships. How are you doing at your job, what are your actions on a daily basis, what are the results that you're getting from your reactions or actions once you do an assessment? Do you have a clear picture of the habits that you have, good or bad?

2: Once you determine those habits, you need to write them down. Make a line on the sheet of paper. On one side you put good habits, on the other side you put bad habits. Now the good habits are going to help you sustain and give you the energy that you need to do or to have to fix the bad habits. Once you identify the good and the bad habits, you go through the bad habits and you write down what needs to be changed and how you're going to change it.

3: This is when you begin to do the work. You take one habit at a time, create a goal of change and get to work. Give yourself a target date to start and a target date that you will be finished by, and at the end of the finish line you will have taken that habit and turned it around and have made it a lifestyle. Now this part is not going to be easy, because you're going to have to change some things about yourself to accomplish the goal, but that's okay. The result will be amazing once you have targeted all these bad habits. These habits have due dates by which they need to be changed. You get to work and you don't stop until it's done. Do not waver, and if you do, you have to start from the beginning. There's a sign that I have on my wall here in the hotel room as I'm finishing this book: ***Stop disappointing yourself, stop making commitments to yourself and not fulfilling your promise to yourself.*** We have a habit of doing that, and that is the one habit that we have to change.

4: You need to journal as you are going through the process of change with the habits. That way you can reread your experiences, which will remind you of the work that you did, so that you don't go back to who you used to be. Journaling is vital to the process, so make sure you either write it down or record a recording in your phone that you can go back and listen to.

5: Once you finish the job of habit changing, pat yourself on the back, give yourself a reward, acknowledge that you've made the change, and share with your closest family or friends and let them know what you've done. That way they can still hold you accountable and they can celebrate with you. Nothing is more exciting than celebrating with friends when you've made a commitment to yourself to change and you finish the job.

It's vital to clearly understand that, if you do not make the attempt to do the work for change, nothing will change in your life. Things will always be the same. Remember, you can't complain about the result you don't get because of the work you don't do.

CHAPTER 6
The Guilt of Change

Change /CHānj/: change, alter, vary, modify, to make or become different. Change implies making either an essential difference often amounting to a loss of original identity or a substitution of one thing for another.

You know this is a very interesting subject for me because change is a word that will forever be a part of my life, and that is because it has been difficult to make changes because of my habits. So I had to make sure that I changed my habits, so things in my life would begin to change. With that being said, change is inevitable when you want to see a difference in your life. But the hard thing about it is, when people notice that you've changed or are making changes, they will try to remind you of who you used to be, because that is what's comfortable for them. This can cause guilt.

People will try to pull you back to who you used to be because that's who they knew you were. When you begin to change, people become very uneasy and then the problem arises. You start to feel guilty because all of the sudden you will find yourself alone.

Now let's talk about that being alone. I want you to understand that sometimes God will clear out all the mess and the people that have no significance in your life, or who are tearing you down, or who are not going the direction that you would like to go, or who are not already there with where you're trying to go. He will clear those people out to make room for your blessings. I need you to understand that you cannot identify change or what you have changed in the midst of chaos and contention. When you have a lot of crazy things going on in your life, your blessing is right around the corner, but you can't find it or identify with it in the midst of chaos. So what you have to do is clear out the path. You've got to clear out the mess so that change can begin to happen, and as it's happening you can identify with it and you will know exactly what it is. And in this process of change, you will become who you want to become, and then you will start to attract who and what you deserve and desire, but that comes with change.

So the guilt in the process is something that you are going to have to control. You're going to have to be unapologetic, intentional, and on purpose to change. Nothing can get in your way. You have to make a decision that you will not feel guilty for the changes that you're about to make in your life right now. You can't allow anyone to make you feel guilty about the changes that you're making in your life that are best for you so that you can live a happy life—not even your mama, your daddy, or anyone else.

When you begin to change your habits and identity, the guilt that can arise stems from your childhood, it stems from your upbringing, it stems from your generation. You are controlled and brought up to believe that you have to stay committed to how you were brought up, with those habits. Any time you make a change, you ruffle people's feathers, because that is not their belief, so you have to be clear that this is what's best for you and your life.

Another part of being guilty or feeling guilty in the process of change is that, when you begin to make a change, your life becomes different, and then at that very moment that you've crossed over it becomes unfamiliar territory. What I mean by this is, you're in a place now where you've done the work to be in that place you've never seen before, so you're going to feel like: Do I really deserve to be in this place of happiness? Do I really feel like I deserve this freedom? Do I really feel like I have choices? And most importantly, do I really feel comfortable with loving myself? So the process is done and now you've crossed over to a new area, so you're thinking to yourself, Oh, I'm here, I've done the work, but I don't recognize anything. That is because you've changed the whole trajectory of your life and soul. For a few moments or a little bit of time, you're going to be guilty or feel guilty about what you've done, what you've lost, what you've eliminated. For the first time in your life you've finished something you committed to for yourself, and you freed yourself of the things that have been weighing you down for so long. So in the process of you feeling uncomfortable with this new space, think about where you've been, what you've suffered from and for how long, how you have sacrificed and put yourself last. That should make you feel like you belong in this area of freedom.

Once you feel that way, you will never turn back. I need you to understand, once you cross over, you need to know you deserve to be there, and don't allow anyone to make you feel guilty about the changes that you've made. Let me tell you, when you make these changes, that's when the narcissists start to show up. They will try to pull you back to who you used to be, but you have to be courageous enough, strong enough and focused, with the ability to tell people, "That is not who I am any longer, that is not the place that I choose to be. I am not going back there, that is not a place for me. I've lived there before, and that's where I was my most miserable." You have to be courageous enough to say that to them and to yourself and believe it.

So you've done the work, you crossed over, and now you have to do the work to stay. The first step is to make a commitment to yourself that you'll never turn back. The second step is, never turn back. The third step: make sure that when you feel weak you connect with the people that are stronger than you. That's going to help you stay in that space. As I've told you in the beginning of this book, everything that we do, all of our actions, or habits, are due to how we were brought up, so when you get in a space based on how you were brought up, this was not the space for you, so it's almost like a rebirth. You are rebirthing yourself to sustain in the space that you belong or believe that you belong.

Changes in action are based on your efforts. You have to be willing to do the work. We have to stop making excuses for not getting the work done. When things get tough, we run. When things get hard, we stop. When we begin to see pushback or feel pushback from others, we feel uncomfortable because they are not happy for us. Those days have to stop right now. Change has to happen, and whatever happens in the process of the change, accept it, deal with it, and keep going. People who understand that the change has to happen will support you, and there are people that won't, but because of the work that you've done with your habits, you will not feel guilty about the change. I promise you you're going to thank yourself later. Change makes everybody uncomfortable, including yourself, but guilt is the last thing you should feel. This is something that you're doing for yourself, not anyone else, and when you finish, your confidence will go from a level 2 to a level 10, and people will start to see you differently. But most importantly, you will start to see yourself differently, and that is a fact.

I remember when I began to make the changes in my life, I had friends that walked away from me, and I had friends that I had to change up on because I realized that those friendships were not for me because of how our relationships developed. In those relationships and friendships, I was always the follower, even though they treated me like my existence wasn't valued. I didn't realize they were skirting their issues by trying to criticize and change me rather than deal with their own issues.

It is very easy for people to try to fix your issues rather than to fix their own, because they're not willing to look in the mirror and take the bandage off of their wounds. So in the process of change I had to let a lot of friendships go, because I realized what our friendship was based on. I thought of myself as less than and I thought I could be more if I was friends with them, which gave them the opportunity to treat me any kind of way and I accepted it. It made them look like the bigger person and they knew it, and that was a weakness of mine.

It's something about the process of change that gives you the strength and the courage to walk away from things that no longer serve you and not accept people just treating you any kind of way. Making decisions for yourself, making the change, creating new habits: this is what happiness is about. The question is: Are you ready for happiness? Because I'm telling you, when you begin to do this work, that's what is going to happen. The result will be you becoming the happiest you've ever been because of the changes that you have made.

In this process, you have to make a commitment that you will never go back to who you used to be because it's comfortable. If it was comfortable, you would not have made the decision to make a change. This is why you're doing the work, because you're sick and tired of being sick and tired.

CHAPTER 7

Forgiveness

What is forgiveness? Psychologists generally define forgiveness as a conscious, deliberate decision to release feelings of resentment or vengeance toward a person or group who has harmed you, regardless of whether they actually deserve your forgiveness. So this is a difficult subject to discuss, because in the process of change I had to go back and relive so many moments to determine what it was that gave rise to the habits that I have today. I had to understand what forgiveness was, and I had to make a decision to forgive those who hurt me, forgive those who abused me mentally and physically. Am I to forgive those who bullied me in high school, am I to forgive those who racially profiled me when I started my career in business?

There was a lot of forgiveness that had to happen, and let me be clear, it wasn't easy. I remember a woman who I worked for as a teenager that clearly used me to make herself look good. She mentally abused me to make me feel like I was nothing so I would become subservient to her, to the point of being disrespected in front of other people, diminishing my value and taking advantage of my unfortunate circumstances. This woman literally told people I was her valet and I was there to assist her with her personal lifestyle. I did everything from cleaning her house, cooking her dinner, taking care of her grandmother, traveling with her, carrying her luggage—the list goes on and on. I had no idea that this was going on, I just thought that this was the right thing to do because of my past. Things got so crazy that at some point I began to run her business, and she used me as a scapegoat to get rid of her boyfriend that she was unhappy with who was running her business at the time. So she put me in the middle of them, and I had to suffer the consequences of his not liking me, from being called names to being talked about, even threats of being physically abused by him or one of his family members. Of course, he didn't act on it and eventually he went away. Then I was stuck running a multi-million-dollar business at the age of 17 years old.

You would think that this would be a great experience. It was, because I learned so much, but what went with it in the process outweighed the learning possibilities. I suffered a lot in those two years. It was painful, I was tired and I was hurt. At some point I was wondering: Why am I going through this? Is this what life is about?

Sitting here writing this, I just realized how much experience I have had over time with running businesses, branding, marketing, managing people, and the list goes on and on, from the age of 16 years old. I am now 54 as I'm writing this book thinking of all of the knowledge that I've gained over the years. The one most important lesson I've learned is forgiveness. These people didn't know any better. You would think they did, but they didn't. One of the things I had to think about was: Why could so many people do wrong and still have a level of success? Why could people hurt people, steal from people, take from people, create a narrative to make themselves look good and other people look bad, but still have a level of success? That is one of the main things that has baffled me in my adult years: why so many people that do so much to hurt other people get away with it, are able to move on with their lives, and feel no remorse. I will never understand, but in me trying to figure that out,

I discovered that these people are people who think about themselves, who feel that they are entitled, and their confidence is through the roof. Regardless of what they do, whether it's wrong or right, they are going to make sure that they come out on top. That is their belief and that belief becomes their reality.

What if you took some of that belief that they have, and do good for yourself and make your dreams your reality? What if you for a moment forgave yourself and were intentional about having a sense of entitlement in a good way, believing that you deserve success, happiness and an amazing life. What if you just believed that for a moment?

Have you ever heard of that saying: *What you think about is what you bring about?* That's what we call manifestation, and once you forgive yourself and others, you free yourself to be able to do all the things that you need to do to make changes in your life and create better habits. It all starts with forgiveness of other people and forgiveness for yourself. That will free you up to create the life that you deserve and that you desire. When you don't know how to forgive, you harbor it, and that is another blockage for your success. So in the process of you taking inventory of all of the habits, all of the things that have happened to you, whether it's good or bad, you do a process of illumination.

One of those things to process is forgiveness. It took me a very long time to forgive the woman who did what she did to me. It took me a very long time to forgive my abusers. It took me a very long time to forgive the people who bullied me in school, and so much more. It's a lot of pain and hurt in the process of forgiveness, but once you get past it, you will be okay, I promise you.

Let's be clear, the people who you need to forgive aren't thinking about you anyway. They've moved on with their lives. You're the only one that's harboring all that has been done to you, and you've allowed it, because of course you didn't know any better. But when you look at it, the people that hurt you don't even think twice, haven't even thought about it again. They just moved on with their lives because that's the way that they operate, that's what abusers do. Your job is to forgive them and move on. I know it's easier said than done, but trust me: when you do it, you will be free. All of the control that they've had over you for years based on what they've done to you will no longer keep you in bondage. You have a choice, so choose wisely.

You don't have to approach these people about these situations and the things that they've done to you. You don't have to speak with them in person. You can speak with them in your mind and spiritually. I know some of you feel like you need to let the person know how you feel or you need to have a conversation with them, but actually you don't have to. This way you won't have to take on the responsibility to determine whether they get your message, realize that they've hurt you, or find yourself in the position of trying to convince them that they ruined your life. You don't need that responsibility. Your responsibility is to take care of you, to move on and get to work on yourself, and that is a part of forgiveness.

It has taken me some time to forgive those who have done what they've done to me. But the more I thought about it and the more that I tried to relive those moments, the more I realized that it was giving them power over me, and I chose to no longer give them that power.

I could tell you more stories of some things that have happened in my past concerning control. I was even in a relationship in my younger years with someone that I thought I had fallen in love with and I was going to spend the rest of my life with. I packed up and moved in with this person. I shared my love, my body, and my life with this individual. Once the dust settled and I became a familiar object, the hunt was over. They chose to look elsewhere for their satisfactions. The feeling I felt in this relationship was the same hurt I felt when I was abused and my abuser got up and walked away after they finished. It was familiar territory and I felt the same pain that I'd always felt. The pain was so familiar that I did not realize that, because of who I was and what I experienced in my past, I continued to attract the same relationships and the same situations over and over again. It had become a pattern. I attracted those things to my life because of who I was, not realizing that I could change it, that I could forgive, and that I could create a new and better life for myself based on the changes. I could create habits that aligned with the direction that I was going in.

One day when I realized that this individual was having an affair outside of our relationship with someone that literally lived in our neighborhood, I accepted it and I dealt with it for months, not realizing that I did not have to stay in that situation. One day I caught them in a hotel. The anger that came over me when I knocked on the door of the hotel room and this individual slammed the door in my face and never came out. I realized that the person that they were with was the priority and I wasn't, but somehow, they made me feel guilty for them having an outside relationship. I picked my head up, walked out of the hotel, got in the car and made a decision that enough was enough. When this individual had to make a business trip, I decided that that was going to be my time to escape. They left that Friday. my things were packed on Saturday morning, and I had moved by Saturday evening into my own apartment.

What was very interesting is that this individual was extremely arrogant and extremely full of themselves, to where they felt no guilt for what they did to me. Somehow or another they turned it around and made me feel like it was my fault that the relationship didn't work when they went outside of our relationship to get satisfaction. And I took on the guilt, and it made me feel like it was my fault and I believed it. I was depressed for months. I only stayed in my apartment for three months and just moved back home to Washington, DC to start all over again like nothing ever happened. My fairytale had turned into a nightmare because I allowed my life to be in somebody else's hands rather than making sure that I took them through a curriculum to teach them how to treat me. I had signs in the beginning but I chose to ignore them.

God will give you a whisper, then he will give you a talking to, and then last but not least he will yell at you and say, "Enough is enough," and because of what I went through in my past and who I had become, I accepted it all. I was miserable and I knew it, and I thought it was the right thing to do. The right thing to do was to get up pack my stuff, and leave. I was young, so I had a lot of energy and nothing could stop me. I had the energy to get up and start all over again and that's what I did. I came back to DC homeless, and within six months I was living in a penthouse downtown. That was an interesting situation itself. I'll get into that another day, but it was a level of success that I'm proud of.

The lesson I learned behind this was that the person who hurt me had a level of confidence and entitlement. No matter what you look like or where you come from, as long as you have confidence and a level of entitlement, you can attract who and what you think you deserve.

Every relationship ended with infidelity or someone going outside of the relationship. So one day I made a decision. I thought to myself, maybe this is what life is about, maybe people can't be loyal or faithful. But that's not for me to figure out, about other people.

What I needed to do was figure out Keith. You see, Maya Angelou couldn't have said it any better: "When people show you who they are, believe them." People will show you who they are in the beginning. You will see signs of who these people are, but it is our fault, because we choose not to believe them. We choose to believe that we are able to fix a person, that we can fix them to be right for us rather than fix ourselves and attract what is right for us! So the lesson learned was when people show up, there's always a representative. Get to know them so you can truly understand what the connection is about.

Forgiveness is hard, and I know that you're carrying the weight of disappointment, regret, and becoming a failure. But it's how you think about it. It's a temporary situation. The disappointment, the regret, and the failure are temporary. What you've got to do is forgive yourself and forgive whoever was a part of the disappointment and start to create a new life for yourself.

You are not obligated to stay in the situation that no longer serves you. The faster you realize that the better off you will be. Don't let situations hold you hostage because of your lack of forgiveness. When you hold on to the guilt, that gives people power to come back and repeat the same thing over and over and over again

CHAPTER 8

Conceptualizing Something Different

con·cep·tu·al·ize /kənˈsep(t)SH(oo͞)əˌlīz/ verb or: conceptualise 1. form a concept or idea of (something).

In my younger years I was a dreamer. I would vicariously live through other people. I would see them live these amazing lives, have happiness in their relationships with their family and their friendships, all the things that I wished I'd had. So when I talk about conceptualize, I'm speaking of dreams. But what you have to do is turn your dreams into your reality. In order to do that, you have to manifest the outcome. It's OK to dream, but the thing is, you have to wake up from your dream to create your reality. A lot of us get stuck in our dreams because it's much easier to dream about it and pretend rather than get up and do the work to create your reality.

Now don't get me wrong, I don't think there's anything wrong with dreaming, but at some point, it's the actions that count. Sometimes you need to write things down and read them over and over again. Write your goals, your values, your mission statement for your life, and then, as you begin to plan it out, you begin to get up, get out, step up, step out, and put some action to the dream.

Some people don't know how to conceptualize something different than their present situation. They don't know how to set their mind to see something different because they're stuck. I was one of those people. I didn't think I could have success. I didn't think I could have happiness because that was unfamiliar territory. But then I started watching and studying other people and realizing they pee and bleed just like I do. I may not have had the same upbringing, but they are no different from me, and so what I had to do was study some of the things that I missed as a child, to become a better me.

I must say, if you're not strong enough to become a better you and you get around people who know that you're weak because of your past situations, they will see you differently and it will devalue your existence. However, as I told you in the beginning of the book, if you're going to choose your friends, choose wisely, and they come forth with no judgment or the ability to take advantage of your vulnerability. So this is when the dreamer in you has to come out. All the things you dream about, you need to write them down. It's time for you to take those dreams, conceptualize them and turn them into your reality. You have to take a few steps, but when you take those steps, it will begin to unfold for you. The first step is to write it down. The second step is to create actions to accomplish the goal. The third step is to do the work, and the last step is to stay consistent. If you do those few things, what you conceptualize will become your reality.

Stop taking your dreams and putting them in the drawer, on the shelf, under the table. It's time to bring them out, because you don't want to go to your grave with regret. Start that job, start that business, buy the new home that you want or that new car. All these things you can do, as long as you understand what it takes to do it and get to work making it happen. You have to have a mindset that anything you want you can have, that it is within reach. You can accomplish that goal. I know people who have done it.

One of the great things about who I have become, one of my attributes, is how I'm able to connect with people. I don't know what it is, but when I set my mind to meeting people, it happens. I am able to do that because I'm genuine, I am intentional. I learned this from Anthony Robbins, Les Brown, and a couple of other people that are connecting with people, that can lead you in the direction that you're going in. It's so important, because they've either done it or got there, or they are going in the same direction that you are. You can't be afraid to step out of your comfort zone. Step up. The worst that can happen is they say no, and no doesn't hurt, it just wasn't your time, so you keep trying or you find somebody else. Eventually you will be connected with the right people to help you get where you need to be.

I'll tell you a little joke. Well, it's not a joke, actually it's my reality. I used to get magazines and I would look at those magazines and I would dream, wishing I could wear those clothes, wishing I could go to those places, wishing I could even drive those nice cars, and every time I set my mind to having those things, or doing those things, it became my reality, because I didn't stop until I got it. That's how I know today that I have to have that same mindset. Somewhere, somehow, I lost that ability to have the strength and the confidence to achieve anything that I wanted, and to be honest with you, I think it was the people that I was hanging around with. We were different, and I lost my zest. I was too afraid to walk away from relationships that did not help me to move forward, because I was afraid to be alone, when actually, that is exactly what I needed to create my success.

There are times when you have to develop new relationships, new connections, and new areas to live and work. You have got to put yourself in those positions for success, take the emotion out of it and get to work.

When I talk about conceptualizing something different, it's about creating the narrative in your head, speaking it out of your mouth and making it your reality. A lot of what we think about is what we do, so for once, try to change the narrative in your head, try to think about something different. When you have negative thoughts, change the narrative. You have to pay attention to the voices in your head. If you don't, you will continue to do the same thing over and over again, because right now you're not healthy enough to switch the thought process you have to build the muscle. You build a muscle in your head by being intentional about focusing on the words in your head. It's not going to be easy, but I guarantee you that if you try it, things will work out differently for you, and you will have a mindset that is unstoppable, unmeasured, and intentional.

I often used to wonder to myself why my upbringing couldn't have been different, and why my relationship with my mom and dad couldn't have been different. For some reason I felt guilty for feeling that way. And then one day I was told by my therapist that I should not feel guilty for the things that were done to me, and I didn't know any better, so I had to get over that. But now that I know it, I don't want to continue to make the same mistakes over and over again. I give myself permission not to feel guilty, and sometimes you have to do that. Often, we look for permission and validation from other people to think that it's going to be OK, to not feel guilty. Again, that is the way we were brought up, that is generational and that's something we have to work beyond.

Family has a tendency to make us feel guilty, but we have to be strong enough to stand up for ourselves and break that generational situation. Sometimes family will even try to make you feel guilty for dreaming, or even your friends, because they may think that's stupid, or it's because they haven't had that experience. It doesn't mean you don't have to, but it's up to you to make a decision to do something different and walk away from the pack.

There's an old story that I always refer back to. There's a difference between an eagle and a chicken. When you see a chicken he's always in a pack, and the one thing that they have in common is they're always pecking and looking down. But when you see an eagle, you see an eagle that is alone, that flies high and looks low. Very seldom do you see them with a lot of other eagles. So my question for you is: are you a chicken or are you an eagle? Are you ready to unapologetically make a new choice for something different so that you can conceptualize a new process?

CHAPTER 9
Never Go Back

So here's the deal: one of the biggest mistakes we all make is that we go back to who we used to be when actually what we should do is look back only to see how far we have come and be reminded of what we never want to experience again. That is another difficult process, because going back and looking back is familiar territory. You gravitate to that area because you don't have to do any work back there, but as you did the work to create the space that you're in now, it takes work to stay and it takes confidence to believe that you deserve to be there.

When I began the trip to make changes in my life, and I crossed over to a better area, it was one of the loneliest times I could ever imagine. I didn't understand why, with all the work I did, all the changes that

I made, I was so lonely and depressed. Then I realized that the old me was gone and a new me was here. It was my time to cultivate new relationships, friendships, and situations for the new Keith that I had created. But it took a long time to realize that because, again, this was unfamiliar territory, so I didn't know what to do. I confidently embraced the change. I stepped up, I stepped out, and I began the process of living in this new life.

Now let's be clear: once you get to this point, there is no turning back at all. You cannot waver, you cannot straddle the fence, you have to be intentional and unapologetic. You cannot allow people to disturb your peace, and you can't keep going back to bad relationships. You can't continue thinking that the situations are right for you because that's all you know. Now you know different, and you have to live in that moment.

I will be honest, I did make some mistakes, and I did go back to who I used to be because I became weak. Let me explain something to you. Every time you go back to who you used to be it becomes twice as hard to get back to who you want to be. That's just like when you want to lose weight or start working out at the gym. When you work out and it becomes consistent, the results are amazing, but when you stop working out you feel the old pain, which becomes worse, and then you try to start it again and it becomes very hard. So save yourself some disappointment and regret and stay on the path to sustaining this incredible person that you've created within yourself.

I was giving a speech one day and a woman asked me a question. "I'm in a relationship and the person that I'm in a relationship with after 10 years decided to move on to someone else because he was no longer attracted to me." Now interestingly enough, we have to respect the man's honesty. He told the truth about why he decided to move on and we cannot hold him responsible because all he was doing was speaking his truth. But the one question I had for this woman, which blew her mind and that of everyone else is in the audience, was: Are you the same person today as you were when you met him in the beginning?

Often, we forget about ourselves in a relationship, we transform into somebody different, we forget to take care of ourselves physically and mentally, and then it begins to show outwardly. What happens with the person that you're with is, you become unrecogniz-able and they seek out what they miss because they're not getting it from you. Now, they can tell you this is what they need and is the problem, or they can make a decision and say that this situation is no longer for them and move on.

Of course, communication is the key, but the question is, have you forgotten about who you are and who you were in order to attract that individual into your life? Why do you think that they made a decision to move on? No, I'm not saying that it's always our fault, but we do need to take these things into consideration. We always take care of others before we take care of ourselves. We always try to make sure everybody is OK before we take care of ourselves, then we become an option, because they know that you're always going to be there.

As an example, when you get on a plane, the first thing they tell you to do in an emergency is to put your mask on first before you put anybody else's on. You are no good to anyone else unless you take care of yourself first. When you take care of yourself, that will give you the willpower to give yourself to someone else. It's called being selfish, and it's being selfish in a good way. You have to realize at some point that you've got to become selfish. Take care of yourself first, love yourself first, love on yourself first, think about yourself first! I know this feels strange to think about yourself first, this is unfamiliar territory, but

I guarantee you that when you focus on yourself it does something to your confidence. It teaches people how to treat you with respect, love, and appreciation. Again, this is another part that takes work, but the results will be amazing when you do this for yourself. To this day I'm learning how to do that—to put me first, love on myself first. Let me tell you something else. When you do these things, you no longer go looking or chasing. You attract to you what is for you, whether it's work relationships, friendships, or situations, you will attract that to you.

As you do these things, you will see that you will never think about going back to who you used to be because who you have become will be so great and so fulfilling. You will become unrecognizable in a good way. People will start to ask you what you are doing, saying, "You look amazing, you're so happy." They won't be able to pinpoint it, but they will know that there is something different, and that's when you have to graciously, and unapologetically, receive the compliment, which is not something we are used to doing. Receive the compliment, know that you deserve it. Receive the compliment, realize that is what you have worked so hard for. Receive the compliment, know that this is your new way of living. You will have your naysayers, the ones who will be negative. That's when you have to build up your strength to walk away and ignore those unhappy people, because they will try to impose their unhappiness on you, and at this point that is not something you're going to settle for. Those days are over. No longer will anyone be allowed to impose their unhappiness on you, and you're going to stop trying to fix those people. That is not your job. There are professionals out there for that. Just because someone needs to be fixed doesn't mean that you have the credentials to fix them to make them right for you.

It's so interesting to me. I always think about something a dear friend said to me, "Dr. Keith, it's always the people giving an opinion that have no credentials to do so, and unfortunately we give them the platform to do it because we don't know any better." That separates the followers from the leaders. It's come to the point where you have to decide that you're no longer a follower, that you are leader of your life, and that you're not going to allow people to impose their beliefs on you, whether they're right or wrong, and what you do and how you conduct your life. You have to be courageous enough to say, "Enough is enough. No more I will allow anyone to disrupt my happiness those days are over." These are the types of things that you're going to have to say to yourself on the regular basis. You're going to have to put up notes and signs that say, "I will no longer allow anyone to disrupt my happiness, I will no longer allow anyone to come into my life knowing they have problems and situations that I know don't agree with or want to be a part of my life."

People pleasing is a sickness that you are going to heal yourself from. Repeat after me:

It is not my job to fix people if they do not have the credentials. It is my job to work on myself so that I attract who and what I deserve and what I desire, and I will no longer make myself a part of something when I'm not prepared for it. I will not impose my problems on people, I will fix myself and do the work.

This is the type of conversation I want you to have with yourself in your head. Get rid of the negativity and put in positive affirmations and get it moving. Never ever go back, it's going to be hard, but you have to make a decision that you're never going to go back. It is your past, and that is exactly what it is: your past. It's now time to create an amazing future and live up to all the possibilities that are available to you. You just have to go out and get them. Do the work, do the work, do the work, and the results will come. Forgive your past, create new habits, conceptualize something different than your present situation, and walk away from what no longer serves you. Never go back!

CHAPTER 10

Bringing It All Together

You've learned so much about me and my process to change. You've learned about breaking the generational habits, you have learned about forgiveness, you have learned about dreaming, you have learned about conceptualizing something different than your present situation, you have learned how to fix it. It's not by making excuses. You have learned that you can never turn back time, you look back only to see how far you have come. You have learned what work you have to do to become who you need to be. You deserve to be in that space of happiness. I am still a work in progress, I still have a lot of work to do, but I'm grateful and thankful for my accomplishments. It took me a very long time to write this book. I know my publisher is shocked that it is finally done, but I had to get past the fear, and the concern about what someone else thinks about me. That is the reason why any time that someone comes to hear me speak, one thing they walk away with is the ability to not concern themselves with what other people think about them. I tell people to write this down and reread it over and over again: "It is none of my business what you think about me." When I adopted this philosophy in my life, I didn't realize how much of an impact it would have on me. For so long I was always concerned about what other people thought about me, what their opinion was and how I could get their approval to accept me, not realizing it was my job to accept myself and then determine who I am willing to accept in my life. I have the power to control that narrative. Often you will forget the power that you have, because that has all been diminished from the past, the relationships and the situations that have devalued your existence. It's hard work, but it will all be worth it.

Take this small book and remember the experiences that I've shared with you and think about it. If I can heal myself, if I can confront my past, with the intent to forgive, you can do the same thing. Remember, it's almost like being an addict: you have to continue to do the work. You can't just walk away and think that it's all over because it's not. Sometimes you're going to be reminded of your past. Sometimes you're going to run into those who are a part of your past. But the great thing is, when you do the work, your response will be different. The hate that you had in your heart, the feelings that you had about people or situations, they will no longer control you, and that is a level of freedom that some people can't even understand. Some of us even want to get revenge, but the best revenge is success and healing. Vindictiveness has no place, nor can be a part of greatness. One day you're going to be able to share your story with others, or you might even just keep it to yourself. I chose to do it because, as I'm writing this book, my decision is to get out, tell my story, speak to the masses, and give them the tools that they need for success.

I have this dream, something that I'm conceptualizing to become a reality, and that's to speak from a great stage. I look out into the audience and I see family. Let me give you the understanding about family. There's a difference between relatives and family. Relatives, you can't choose them, but family you can. Always remember, you have choices. In this dream I see myself coming down some steps that kind of remind me of Luther Vandross. I don't know if you've ever seen him in concert. If you have not you need to go to YouTube and watch him perform. His stage presence was always incredible. I had this dream of coming down some steps that are going to be lighting up to this amazing pumped-up music that is going to get the audience pumped, ready, and excited about what I'm about to teach them. That has been a dream of mine, and that is one of the reasons why I decided to sit in this hotel and finish this book. This book has been in development for over three years. I realized that I was unhappy with this unfinished business. I was unhappy with my energy, I was unhappy with my success, and I had to adopt a level of determination to get this done no matter how uncomfortable it was.

As I'm writing this, I'm at the end of this book and I'm ready to send it over to my publisher. This was the day that I made a decision that changes needed to be made. I told you I was a work in progress. For so long I have been disappointing myself, for so long I've been making promises to myself and did not keep them, for so long I've been telling everybody that this was going to be done, it was no longer a dream; it became a lie. Some people didn't believe this book was coming out, some people even asked for a refund because they got tired of waiting. The embarrassment of that and dis-appointing myself was another situation to take on, and how I handled this whole situation just based on my past experiences. I didn't think I was worthy of the success. I didn't think that anything would come out of this, but then I realized if I just do this one thing, that will start the beginning of something huge. That is, my dreams would become a reality, and that the steps are being taken to sustain and to live in my passion. I no longer compare myself to other people. And I'm very mindful of some of the people that I have around me, who under the radar compete with me, and they never want me to do better than them, but that's okay. They'll come around, and they will understand that we're in this together. It's not about who does better than everyone else. It's about the outcome and how many people you can help in the process.

The process for me finishing this book today was as follows: 1) I made a decision. 2) I made a plan. 3) I blocked out interruptions and distractions. 4) I stayed focused. 5) I gave myself a timeline. 6) I journaled the process. 7) I followed the timeline to the T. 8) I wrote affirmations and posted them around my hotel room. 9) I exercised on my breaks to sustain a great deal of energy. 10) I celebrated my wins. This is the process I used to finish everything in my life!

Everything has to have a plan, almost like having a map. You can't get there unless you have direction and a plan, so I'm asking you today to sit down and take inventory of your past and determine if your past has anything to do with who you are today. Understand, you have the ability, if you want to change at all and not let your past dictate your future. All you have to do is start. Once you get started it becomes easier and easier and you're going to love the results. I guarantee you things will begin to unfold that you never ever imagined.

A lot of what you see in successful people is their ability to fix themselves, create a life that they've always dreamed of and execute the work that it takes to sustain it. You can be one of those people, to step up and realize that *your present situation is not your final destination.* When you get to your final destination, you're going to look back briefly, quickly, and see where you've come from. That will give you the energy to create more success for yourself based on your past and what you've been through that has given you the willpower.

If you've been through all of that you can do anything. If you can suffer through the pain, you can do anything. If you can be abused and live through it, you can do anything. Take all that you've been through, roll it up in a ball, serve it to yourself and take all of that and create this incredible life.

If you're reading this book, that means you're alive and you can make a difference right now. All it takes is a decision. Don't waste another moment. It's not too late. It's never too late. Step up, step out and make it happen.

Thank you so much for reading this small, sweet book of my experience in life. Reach out to me and let me know what you think about all of this. Let me know if this relates to you or if you've been through any of the same things. Let me know how this has helped you. I am grateful and I'm thankful for you. Know that you and I are a work in progress.

Love,

Keith

Printed in the USA
CPSIA information can be obtained
at www.ICGtesting.com
LVHW070103291023
762360LV00013B/659